T0086284

TIPS & TRICKS
for VIPS
(Visually Impaired Persons)

Ruth McKinsey

WESTBOW
PRESS®
A DIVISION OF THOMAS NELSON
& ZONDERVAN

Copyright © 2016 Ruth McKinsey.

All rights reserved. No part of this book may be used or reproduced by any means, graphic, electronic, or mechanical, including photocopying, recording, taping or by any information storage retrieval system without the written permission of the author except in the case of brief quotations embodied in critical articles and reviews.

Scripture taken from the New King James Version. Copyright 1979, 1980, 1982 by Thomas Nelson, inc. Used by permission. All rights reserved.

This book is a work of non-fiction. Unless otherwise noted, the author and the publisher make no explicit guarantees as to the accuracy of the information contained in this book and in some cases, names of people and places have been altered to protect their privacy.

WestBow Press books may be ordered through booksellers or by contacting:

WestBow Press
A Division of Thomas Nelson & Zondervan
1663 Liberty Drive
Bloomington, IN 47403
www.westbowpress.com
1 (866) 928-1240

Because of the dynamic nature of the Internet, any web addresses or links contained in this book may have changed since publication and may no longer be valid. The views expressed in this work are solely those of the author and do not necessarily reflect the views of the publisher, and the publisher hereby disclaims any responsibility for them.

Any people depicted in stock imagery provided by Thinkstock are models, and such images are being used for illustrative purposes only. Certain stock imagery © Thinkstock.

ISBN: 978-1-5127-4402-6 (sc)
ISBN: 978-1-5127-4403-3 (e)

Library of Congress Control Number: 2016908640

Print information available on the last page.

WestBow Press rev. date: 05/31/2016

I encourage caregivers of visually impaired persons to read this book with them. You will both benefit. Please go to the end of the introduction of this book to see instructions to access *free* MP3 audio files of the book, read by the author. I want to make sure complete access of this book is available to the blind or partially sighted individual.

When you're feeling powerless,
don't let anyone tell you there is nothing you can do.
Listen, learn, grow, share, give back, and thrive.

Contents

Acknowledgments and Dedications

My name is Ruth McKinsey, and I have enjoyed every minute of my volunteer work with blind and partially sighted adults for over thirty years. I worked with the Stanislaus Association of the Visually Impaired for many years and have served on the board of directors of the Visually Impaired Persons Support Center in Modesto, California, for twelve years.

I would like to thank my husband, Marty, for not complaining while I have invested many hours in the workings of a nonprofit organization that is dedicated to the welfare of visually impaired citizens. He has been a great inspiration and a help to me and others as we work together to provide these services to those who live in the community we both grew up in and love.

I would like to thank my daughter, Bree Noble, for teaching me so much about living and thriving with a visual impairment. If it were not for her, I probably would never have become involved with the blind community. Born with congenital glaucoma, she has dealt with partial vision her whole life. At eighteen, she unfortunately lost complete sight in her right eye and was forced to adjust once again. Because of her "I can do it" attitude, she earned two college degrees in four years. At thirty, she was able to have cataract surgery, which restored some vision in her left eye. At forty-three, she is happily married, has two beautiful girls, has worked successfully as an accountant, and is now CEO of her own music business: WOSradio.com. She is still legally blind and will never drive a car, but that hasn't stopped her from living a very productive and fulfilled life.

When she was growing up, there was little support in our community for anyone with such a disability. She did have some help in school, but we had no guidance from any organization as to what types of training or support was available to us. We did get some monetary assistance from our local Lions Club to help purchase a reading machine when she was about eight years old. The Lions Club is one organization that specifically reaches out to help with the needs of blind people of all ages.

I would also like to thank the founders of the Visually Impaired Persons Support Center in Modesto. The champions who had a vision and acted upon it are Jim and Pat Syvertsen, who had the idea for the center, optometrist Brian Elliott, OD, who already had a support group going for people dealing with diseases that cause blindness, and Pat Gillum and John De La Mora. These were the initial board members who took on the daunting project of forming the 501(c)(3). They were able to procure a physical location for one dollar a year from the city, which allowed the center to provide services to the blind community for free, funded by private donations only. If it were not for them, the organization would not exist.

I would also like to thank the devoted and oh-so-talented staff members of VIPS for their dedication and professionalism. Most of them have a visual impairment and have worked harder than most to overcome the obstacles they have encountered while reentering the workplace to become a vital part of the organization. I commend each one of them for their accomplishments and for providing the highest level of excellent training to all of their clients.

A big thank-you goes out to Chris Hansen, blinded at birth, for his contribution of chapter 17. He is a talented writer and loves a good joke. I am very pleased to include his contributions to the chapter on laughter. Keeping a good sense of humor is essential in getting past the pain in many situations. Losing your sight can be devastating, but losing your sense of humor about it can be fatal. I know you will enjoy his contribution to the book.

Finally, I would like to thank the many clients who have passed through VIPS's doors on their way to redirecting their lives to personal independence. The people I have encountered and come to love are among the bravest people I know. I have watched them grow in confidence, be filled with hope for their future, become more self-aware, develop a deeper faith in their Creator, be more accepting of others, give charity to others, and grow in humility, generosity, and courage. And the list goes on. I have learned much more from them than they will ever learn from me.

I dedicate this book to all those who are overcoming their blindness with a desire to create a vision for their future and the tenacity to put a plan in motion to achieve greatness in spite of adversity. We all have difficulty in life, but what is really important is how we use those hardships to our advantage and grow in character through them. If you are reading this book because you are losing, or have lost your sight, I hope this book will aid in your journey in reestablishing your personal independence. God speed, and may he bless you abundantly.

Introduction

I have gleaned most of my tips and tricks working with clients who have come through the Visually Impaired Persons Support Center (VIPS) in Modesto, California. I have been very fortunate to become friends with many of these clients and have enjoyed watching them blossom from the various trainings they receive at the center. I am a witness of how a life can change when given the right tools to work with. The organization was established in 2003 to provide services to partially sighted and blind citizens of Stanislaus County, and since not everyone lives within traveling distance of this center, I have written this book to share its wisdom with people who are losing or have already lost their sight.

Let me share a little about what the center actually does for its clients. VIPS takes pride in providing professional training in several essential areas. The first of these is technical training in adaptive technology. This includes computers fitted with several types of software created to assist legally blind individuals to continue to use their personal computers. Some programs simply magnify the words as large as needed for each student; VIPS uses ZoomText. There is also Jaws, which audibly reads all the text on the screen to the student. With these programs, students learn to do any type of word processing and navigate the Internet, including email and social media.

The technical instructors also provide training in smartphone usage and other devices that scan text and translate it to Braille or simply read it to the student audibly.

VIPS also provides independent living skills in its full-service kitchen and workroom. In this program, students are taught to prepare and cook their favorite foods, organize and maintain an efficient kitchen and household, and even learn to iron and sew if they desire these skills. These instructors also teach literary Braille.

A third service VIPS provides is orientation and mobility training. These classes teach how to use a cane and how to take busses, trains, and planes by yourself. This is a vital training that will help you become independent again and be able to go out of your home with confidence. This training also includes how to walk safely with a sighted guide.

A delightful part of this organization is the support groups. When people lose their sight, it is a huge adjustment and many go from being active in the workplace to being isolated in their homes. Both partially sighted persons and their caregivers are invited to the weekly meetings to help them gain confidence to learn to adapt to their new, uncertain, and unfamiliar world.

In 2012, many of the support group members participated in writing a book about adjusting to blindness called *The Little House That Cares*. It gives a lot of hope to anyone who has just received the news that he will soon lose his sight or to those who have already experienced complete blindness. There are seventeen stories of vision loss and life recovery that will give any person dealing with vision loss hope for their future.

The group had a wonderful time writing that book, and I was privileged to compile all the stories and edit the book too, with a lot of help from a few generous, retired schoolteachers. I have seen how it has helped people get a better understanding of what happens in the life of a person who suddenly loses his sight. Each story is gripping and insightful.

Each week the support group attendees share tips and tricks to help the newcomers cope with their blindness. I thought it was about time to share many of them with those who cannot train in a center like VIPS or be a part of a support group.

I have learned so much from the brave clients who have come to the center for guidance and want to pass on their wisdom to anyone who may be going through the same experience. They are eager to share what has helped them the most and what has been a hindrance to their progress.

This book is written for anyone who has just lost part or all of his sight and is wondering what the next step should be. I hope you will be blessed by my efforts to guide you in the right direction.

I would be terribly remiss if I did not offer an audio version of this book. If you have purchased this book, please go to www.tipsandtricksforvips.com for full instructions on how to download a *free* MP3 audio book. You can also purchase my other publications at www.valleyartisans.net.

1

Taking Action after My Vision Loss:
What Do I Do Now?

You may have recently heard the words "You are losing your vision, and there is nothing we can do about it." Or you have already experienced the reality of permanent vision loss. I understand that losing something you have depended upon your whole life has just been taken away from you and you are more than likely expected to keep on functioning like everything is normal, visible, and intelligible.

But you can't see; you don't feel normal, and many things are no longer understandable like they were when you could see them. It can be a devastating realization that you wish would just go away, but in all probability, it isn't going to go away.

You need to understand that now that things are different, you will need to conduct your life differently. You can do the things you were doing before your vision loss; you will just be doing them in new ways. Don't get stuck, thinking that your life is over. It is far from over but there are several stages you will probably go through as you adjust to your blindness. In the support groups, they talk about these stages frequently. You will almost always experience some or all of these stages.

Janet, a VIPS manager, suffers from retinitis pigmentosa. She frequently leads the group and can certainly empathize with most of the attendees. Her story is written in *The Little House That Cares,* where she also talks about going through different stages of grief.

She points out four major stages of grief associated with any loss, including blindness. She makes it very personal and relates it to vision loss specifically.

1. **Denial**. At first, you will more than likely go through a denial stage. You just can't believe that this sight loss is permanent. You may even be saying to yourself, "This is a modern society with new cures discovered every day. I am sure one will come along soon for my condition. I'll just get another opinion from a better doctor and then he will save my sight." This reaction is pretty typical of most people who are given a diagnosis of any type that is life changing. Change is a scary thing, and sometimes we just don't want to accept the things that change brings.

2. **Anger.** It is never fun to go through this stage, but more than likely, it will rear its ugly head. You may be thinking, *It just seems that someone ought to be to blame for my misfortune.* Unfortunately, the rain falls on the

just and the unjust and none of us is immune to trials in this world. Don't feel guilty if you have feelings of anger; just get it out and get on with your plan for dealing with the problem at hand.

3. **Depression.** This is a cliff you may fall over, for a time. Understanding the permanence of your condition and your lack of control of the situation may cause you to succumb to despair. We have seen many people come into the support groups with their heads bent low and their countenances hopeless. But after they get to know others who have walked in their shoes and made it up the daunting mountain in one piece, they begin to lose their sense of despair. Obviously, you should speak with your doctor if the depression continues for a long period of time, but really, the best cure for a solitary pity party is to invite some friends in to change the mood of the party. At VIPS, they always say, "Go ahead. Feel sorry for yourself, for a short time. Just as long as you *don't continue* to feel sorry for yourself and get stuck there."

4. **Acceptance.** This is when the healing can start; when you and your family can settle on the fact that things will be different from now on. At this point, you can start to put together a plan to learn how to deal with your blindness head-on.

It is imperative that you stay in close communication with your eye doctor to understand your condition and become aware of what you should do in case of any changes in your eyesight. There are many eye conditions that can cause damage rapidly if you don't take action and see your doctor immediately, so always be vigilant about your eye care.

Losing your sight isn't an easy thing to accept, and it may take you a while to accept the diagnosis. Once you have, there are steps you can take to make the adjustment easier for you as well as your family members and friends.

That is why this book was written. I want you to have the advantage of getting the ball rolling toward a brighter future. Although you may feel you have a dim future ahead of you, I want to give you the tools to regain control over your destiny and the independence you have been accustomed to in your previous, sighted world. I can assure you that it is not only possible but likely that you will be able to flourish in spite of your loss of sight.

Dr. Brian Elliott sits on the board of the Modesto VIPS center and sees most of the patients who come through the doors. I asked him for a few tips in relation to what the first steps should be after your diagnosis. Here are a few of his suggestions for those who are going in for their initial exam to determine just how much sight they have and what aids might be available for them.

- When you come to your initial examination, you will want to bring all your glasses, magnifiers, and any other portable devices you use on a daily basis.
- Think about specific tasks that you find difficult due to your vision loss (i.e., reading the newspaper and operating the microwave) and bring them to the attention of your doctor. General statements like "I

just want to see better" are not usually helpful toward meeting your goals.

- Bring examples of reading materials you wish to read.
- Write down questions you want to ask before your visit.
- Bring previous eye history information (names of current eye care specialists, past eye surgeries, etc.).
- Expect to be dilated at each visit.
- Expect an initial examination time of one and a half or two hours.
- Expect that you may need more than just glasses to perform daily tasks.
- Expect that you may need specific training to deal with the effects of vision loss.

If you have no sight left and don't think you need an exam, remember that you still need to keep up with your doctor visits. Glaucoma, for instance, can continue to affect a blind eye and become very painful. The pressure can climb even after complete blindness, and there are ways to deal with it to give you relief. I have even heard that a very low pressure can cause pain and this also can be relieved with a medical procedure. Listen to your doctor.

2

Steps to Making Adjustments to My Blindness

In order to succeed at anything, you need a plan. There should be steps to an end, or you will lose your way in the process. I have tried to put together a sensible and proven plan to help you arrive at your intended goal; living an independent life again. This is not a one, two three steps and you are done type of plan. This plan includes successfully dealing with your disability in a satisfactory manner that helps you maintain your independence and live an abundant life.

Where Should I Start?

To start out, ask your eye doctor if he is aware of any nonprofit organizations in your area dedicated to helping people with vision loss. You could also call your local Lions

Clubs or public service organizations to see if they are aware of local help for the blind and visually impaired.

Check with information (411) to see if they have any "vision loss" organizations listed. If they do, call them and make an appointment to visit their facility and become acquainted with the services they offer. Unfortunately, they are usually only located in highly populated cities, such as San Francisco or Seattle. If you do have one in your area, they can help you start the process of contacting your state department of rehabilitation to set your training program in motion.

For many, this book is a good start. Also, *The Little House That Cares* is a good source of encouragement. You can order this by calling The Visually Impaired Persons Support Center at 209- 522-8477.

If you don't have a blind center in your area, contact your state government's department of rehabilitation. It will have some training available to help you adjust to your vision loss and will arrange classes in the nearest facility to you. If you want to keep working, it may be able to help you obtain adaptive equipment. If you feel that would be too difficult and you qualify to go on disability, you will receive money from the state. Each state is different, so please contact yours for that information.

Once you have taken these steps, and you are waiting for the government to get the ball rolling for you, use this book to get ahead of the game. You will find tips and tricks for every area of your life in the next chapters.

3

Educating Family and Friends about My Blindness

One of the things that can be quite hard is getting your family and friends to understand that you cannot see like you could before. They tend to play the denial game and don't want to accept your limitations, just like you didn't want to accept them either.

Everyone with a visual impairment experiences different levels of sight. Some see nothing but darkness; some see only shadows; some see nothing but white (possibly from a cataract). Some have holes in their vision or only see small patches in front of them, and some may have no peripheral vision at all so it feels like they are looking through the center of a doughnut. Each case is unique.

Your loved ones might watch you fall over a coffee table but then notice that you are able to see a piece of white thread on a dark carpet. This may cause them to think you are not being honest about your vision loss.

The truth is you could have excellent vision, but only in one tiny spot within your focus. This does not mean it is safe for you to cross a busy street without the assistance of a sighted guide or a cane. Your loved ones need to understand just how your eyes are affected and what that means for you to travel safely.

You may want to look up your particular disease on the Internet and then show them the effect this disease has on your eyes. It may help them to understand a bit better. Often your local blind center will have demonstration cards that they can hold over their eyes to show just how a person sees with a particular eye condition. It is very shocking to have a loved one look through this device and realize just what you are seeing on a daily basis.

Remind them that they can't direct you by saying things like "You can find it? It's right over there." They also need to understand that they can't leave cupboard doors open or the dishwasher door down where you can trip over it. If they move the furniture, they need to tell you or move it back in place.

These might seem like minor things, but getting everyone in your household to understand that things will be a bit different for you and them from now on is very important.

Invite them to a support group if there is one available in your area. Have them read *The Little House That Cares* to try to understand how others have accepted the vision loss of their loved ones. This book includes stories by several people who have lost their sight and several caregivers who have walked side by side with them through their adjustment to their new way of life without sight.

Tip: Don't get discouraged! There is a big learning curve here, and you need to be aware that just when they are comfortable with understanding just what you do see, your vision might change again. Frustration levels will be high on both sides.

Tip: Having a sense of humor is a great asset. When you mistake a dog bone for a cookie and pop it into your mouth, don't be embarrassed and slink into the corner; offer one to the rest of your guests to see if they might like them too.

Trick: Share your magnifier with those around you so they can see details on a dollar bill that they never knew were there. Make what you are learning to do interesting to others. (This is a trick my daughter used when she had to use a dome magnifier as a child in school.)

4

When Should I Play the "Blind Card"?

Playing your "blind card" means taking advantage of an offer or benefit available to you because you are visually impaired. None of us likes to appear helpless or weak, but when you lose your sight, there are just some things you can't do the way you could when you were fully sighted. Here are a few times you should take advantage of what is available to you as a legally blind person.

- The state offers you a "handicapped" placard for your car because of your disability. You can apply on line at http://www.dmv.ca.gov/portal/wcm/connect/ aebb95cd-c20a-49bd-bc13-dd74120044fc/reg195. pdf?MOD=AJPERES. More than likely, you don't drive, but when family or friends take you places, they can park near the front of the store. A big parking lot with lots of cars pulling in and out can be a very hazardous place. My daughter was almost hit by a backing car in a parking lot. It is much better for you to be near the front of the store.

Tip: Notice where the marked-off, open area is next to the handicapped parking space. This extra space is actually created for wheelchair access from a van. Have your driver back into the space, if the open area is on the left side. This will give you more room to exit and enter the vehicle without stepping into traffic too quickly.

- The phone company offers free (411) information on your home phone. Now that you can't use a phone book or see the numbers on the phone, take advantage of the free (411). You can also get a free phone with large numbers if that helps you. Call your local carrier to see what it requires to get the service free.

- If you visit a museum, ask for a free audio headset that explains the exhibits to you. Most facilities will provide this type of headset. One example would be the zoo.

- If you can get a reduced price on a train, bus, or plane ticket because of your disability, take it. When making a reservation, ask if there are any discounts for disabled persons and what they require as proof of a disability.

5

The Need to Stay Connected

Often when people lose most or all of their sight, they tend to withdraw from friends and sometimes even family members. It is very important to continue to socialize with your current friends and to find a way to make new friends. This is where a support group is very valuable. When you attend a support group meeting, you will meet others who are going through the same thing you are going through. They may have been dealing with it longer than you and are then able to give you encouragement to not give up.

Make sure you have the phone numbers of other people in the group. If you are having a bad day, you might want to call them for support, or if you are having a great day, call them with encouragement.

Often we see people come into the group for the first time—hanging their head, unresponsive, and depressed with feelings of complete despair. Once they get to know the group and gain confidence because of what they see others accomplishing, they learn to interact with the group and feel better about themselves.

Meeting People for the First Time

Meeting new people can be awkward, even if you don't have a vision problem, but when you are introduced to someone and you can't see them, it becomes a little more stressful. The best advice I have for you is to take the initiative when it comes to meeting new people. Don't wait for them to approach and thrust out their hand to shake yours; they will probably feel uncomfortable because they don't know how much you can see and if you will be able to see that they have their hand extended. They may think about grabbing your hand, but then that seems rude. Regardless, sometimes they will grab you and that can be startling, so you may as well be the one to initiate the handshake.

Why not lead off the conversation by introducing yourself and extending your hand first? Obviously, they will see your friendly gesture and shake your hand comfortably. Don't be a fainting flower. Be bold and show them that you are still you and you are interested in meeting new people. If the other person is also blind, let them know that you would like to shake their hand to get to know them better.

It will take practice, but learning to recognize people by their voice is essential. When you can no longer count on your sight, lean on your other senses to help fill in the gaps. Be a better listener and sharpen your memory so you can remember voices of the people you meet. Maybe they wear a perfume or aftershave that will help you recognize them before they even say a word.

Tip: By shaking hands, you can learn a lot about people. You can tell their approximate age by their skin and even what type of work they do. Is their hand like a farmer's hand or a banker's hand? We have a friend who is a cow milker and he just about crushes my bones every time he shakes my hand. He doesn't know his own strength. I just had to ask him what he did for a living the first time I shook his hand, and it led to a wonderful conversation. He is much gentler when we meet now.

Tip: You may want to keep a small recorder with you to keep track of the names of the people you meet. If you have set an appointment to get together with them, you can record it and have it for future reference. You may want to record their email address or phone number in order to keep in contact with them. (This tip was demonstrated many times by Ron in support group.) You could also do this on a smartphone.

Tip: Keep your face forward and don't put your head down or tilted up into the air. Keep it level with their face. This will make them more comfortable, even though you can't really see their face well. (This tip was given to my daughter by a blind professional singer and piano player who actually hired a dance choreographer to help him with stage presence. When he was performing, you would have no idea that he was completely blind as he looked toward the audience frequently with a smile on his face.)

Tip: Almost every visually impaired person I meet tells me that humor is the most important factor when in any new type of social situation. Meeting people is certainly one of those times.

Tip: Old friends may approach you and expect you to know who they are. You could say something like this when you encounter an old friend who may not be aware of your vision loss: "I may have lost most of my sight, but to me, you look just like I remember you."

Tip: Don't be embarrassed to admit that you don't recognize someone. If someone approaches and talks to you and you don't know who it is, simply say, "I'm sorry; who am I speaking to?" Explain that your vision isn't what it used to be and you wish you could greet people by name, but it just isn't possible. Let them know that when *they* forget your name, you won't think less of *them*.

6

Keeping in Touch with the World

Reading the newspaper and getting connected on the Internet are great ways for you to keep up with what is going on in the world. Although you may not have the ability to visually read the paper, books, or the computer screen, there is no reason to think that you cannot keep in touch with what is going on in the world. There are lots of ways to access these sources.

Of course, getting training in adaptive technology would be your number one source. VIPS center makes sure that the students are able to access the Internet, which includes Facebook, email, and all the other sources of daily news. This is training that your department of rehab would set up for you to start.

Many sources are available through the Library of Congress. You can fill out an application for recorded books that are absolutely free to you with a confirmation from your doctor that you are legally blind. They will even provide you with a digital player to play them. You can also get just about any magazine and also newspapers. If you love to read, don't stop now. You can order classic books that will give you endless hours of enjoyment. (See resources in chapter 21.)

Tip: Most books are available on the cloud now so they are accessible through computers, Kindle, pads, and phones. Check out Bookshare.com as another source for free books.

7

Should I Consider Getting a Guide Dog?

The difference between using a white cane and using a guide dog is the white cane will find an obstacle in your path whereas the guide dog simply guides you around it. You may not even be aware that an obstacle is in your path when the dog guides you around it. A pothole is an example of this.

Just because you are legally blind, it doesn't mean that you should have a guide dog. The actual percentage of blind individuals with a guide dog is quite small—maybe 1 percent. Although you don't have to purchase a dog, they cost around $65,000 to raise and train before they are ready to be paired with an owner. The money is provided by private individuals and businesses who are interested in aiding the blind with a gift of a guide dog. You have to go to guide dog training for several weeks to get to know your dog and find out if you are a good match.

You also have to be quite mobile already. This means that you have to be able to get around your community by yourself, with the aid of a cane, and you take the initiative to do this frequently. When you get a dog, you have to work the dog daily, so you have to be an active person who is physically able to exercise your dog.

You also have to be an advocate for the guide dog program. Believe it or not, there are still many people who do not understand what a guide dog does. They may think that the dog simply knows where you want to go and he or she leads you there. Nothing could be farther from the truth. You need to know where you are going, but the dog will be a great asset when it comes to crossing streets or encountering hazards on the sidewalk. They will guide you around a hole in the street, stop if a car is coming toward you, hesitate before a step, etc.

Many people are still not even aware that it is legal to take a guide dog into a restaurant, hotel, or a public place where ordinary dogs are not permitted.

I just have to tell you what happened to a friend of mine who owns a beautiful dog named Velour. I need to point out that she is always polite and realizes that she is an advocate for the blind community, so she always tries to be pleasant when dealing with the public.

She and a friend were at an open-air flea market for the afternoon. The guard approached my friend and told her that she was not allowed to have a dog on the property. He pointed to the sign showing a dog with a slash through it, indicating that no dogs were allowed. She proceeded to tell him that

Velour was a guide dog so it was okay for him to be there. He retorted with, "Lady, you cannot have that dog here!"

She countered with the same answer, "She is a *guide dog!*" She told him that his supervisor should be called and went about her shopping. Soon she ran into him again.

"Lady, you need to get that dog out of here!" he insisted.

"It is a guide dog!" she said again, sternly.

He answered her back, rather abruptly, "I don't care if it is a *guy* dog or a *girl* dog; you still can't have it here!

I kid you not! This really happened, and it just shows that even those in authority don't always understand what the rules are for service dogs. You have to help educate the community about their purpose.

You are not supposed to let people pet or feed them when they have a harness on, but that is really hard to enforce when in public. Everyone loves a pretty dog and wants to pet them.

Please don't get me wrong; a guide dog can be a wonderful comfort and a great asset to a legally blind person. I know people who wouldn't think of being without a guide dog, but they do become like family and when they pass, it can be very devastating to the owner. In general, they have to retire after about five years because they just stop wanting to guide and, because they are getting older, they are just not as interested in guiding as they used to be.

I just want you to be aware of lots of things to think about before you consider partnering up with a canine.

- Are you proficient at getting around your town without a sighted guide and correctly using a cane? The guide dog providers will not give you a dog if you don't know how to navigate your surroundings. You have to be mobile and able to exercise your dog every day.

- Are you a dog person? Caring for an animal is a big responsibility, and it is even harder once you have lost your sight.
- Does your family like animals? Does anyone have an allergy to dogs? Making your family miserable isn't a good idea.
- Are you able to exercise and work the dog every day? These dogs are on a schedule. You will have to rise at the same time each day to feed him and take him out to relieve himself. You will wait until he eliminates and then dispose of it immediately. If you don't, you will have to deal with stepping in it later. Guide dog school teaches you all of these tips.
- You also have to walk with the dog a certain number of hours a day; they are working dogs and they need to work each day. They will get lazy and forget how to guide.
- Are you able to pay for and take your dog to the vet on a regular basis? Some vets will give discounts for guide dogs, but you would be responsible to find one that does.
- Are you able to keep up with the household maintenance, such as cleaning up dog hair and dirt tracked in by a dog? Most guide dogs are Labs or German shepherds, and they both shed. I recently took care of a yellow Lab and literally had to vacuum twice a day to keep up with the shedding. A month later, I am still finding light dog hair in my carpet. Does that work for you?

On the other hand, if you are a dog person and you love animals and the companionship they can provide, there is nothing like a guide dog. The relationships I have seen between guide dogs and blind owners are very special. You should definitely contact Guide Dogs for the Blind (http://welcome. guidedogs.com/) or another organization that provides guide dogs to the blind and see what they might have in store for your future. It could be the start of a wonderful relationship that will benefit you tremendously.

Better yet, get to know someone who owns a guide dog and talk to them about the benefits and disadvantages, if there are any, to having a dog. Be wise and think of all the reasons you should, or shouldn't, have a guide dog.

8

Traveling with a Sighted Guide

More than likely, you will not have a guide dog right away, if at all. When you venture out of your home, you will probably either use a cane, if you have been trained to use it, or have someone go with you to help guide you. This is called having a sighted guide. Believe it or not, there are a few very important things you need to learn, so you can teach your sighted guide—if you don't want to be dragged through the streets like a child. It is important that you learn these techniques and then teach them to whomever you are using as a guide.

The more time you spend walking with a sighted guide, the better you will be at it. At first, you will tend to pull back and not trust the people you are being guided by, so you will need to learn to trust them by teaching them what makes you feel secure.

Most partially sighted or blind people have a preference of what side they would like the guide to be on. For instance, if you are right handed, you might want them to be on your left side so you can use your right hand to hold a handbag, briefcase, water bottle, cane, or whatever you might have with you. Here is a suggestion of how you could talk to your sighted guide:

- "May I show you how I would like to be guided?"
- "I prefer to be on your right (or left) side, so I can still use my dominant hand. Is that okay?"
- "If you will simply bend your right (or left) arm at the elbow, I will grasp the back of your arm just above your elbow. I won't need to hold it tightly, but just enough to take direction from you."
- "When you come to a curb or a change in the surface level, please let me know it is coming. If you go slowly down or up a step, I will be able to sense the change in levels and follow right along with you. If we come to stairs, up or down, let me know approximately how many there are and if we are going up or down. Believe it or not, going down is more difficult for me. Let me hold the banister on my free arm side for my own security, and yours."

If you can plainly and simply talk to your sighted guide like this, you will both be on the same page before you start your walk. It will become easier and easier for you to trust and walk smoothly with any sighted guide if you practice this tip.

9

Traveling Safely by Myself

Safety is your main concern when traveling by yourself. This is true as you travel around your own home, in your neighborhood, or to another city. This is why it is vitally important that you learn to use a cane and take it with you when you travel. There are straight canes and folding canes. The straight cane can stand in a corner of your home until you need it to navigate around your home, and a folding cane can be taken with you when you go out in public. Use it to navigate and then fold it up and store it in your backpack or handbag when you arrive at your destination.

The best way to learn how to use your cane is to have mobility lessons from a certified mobility teacher. This is one of the most important classes at VIPS. Every person who has lost significant sight should take this class.

Tip: Keep a cane in your home to help you navigate through your own house and yard. If you live alone, you will probably keep everything in its place, but if you have others living in your household, they will more than likely leave in your path things that could become safety hazards for you.

When away from home, having a cane not only helps you feel your way around in strange surroundings, it also indicates to others that you may need some assistance. People cannot be blamed if they run into you because you don't see them. They need to understand that you can't see them. Don't be worried if you are not completely blind. Use it anyway and simply explain that you have holes in your vision that keep you from being able to navigate without a cane. People will understand and are usually happy to help.

Occasionally, you will get the skeptic who says, "I saw you pick up that glass on the table; you aren't really blind." That is your cue to give them an education about blindness. Remember you are an ambassador for the whole blind community, so be pleasant and help them understand your situation. You may be the only blind person they have ever come in contact with and they really have no idea what being legally blind really means.

If you are new to an area or you are planning to spend time in a new area, there are steps you should take to make sure you will be able to navigate confidently when you are alone.

Start out by taking a sighted guide with you to this place. Let's say you are going to attend a junior college. Have your class schedule with you and the locations of your classes. Have the sighted guide lead you to all of the classrooms, the dining area, the bookstore, the restrooms, the gym, and any other areas you will be frequenting. This will give you a chance to understand any hazards you may encounter, such as stairs, detours, blocked sidewalks, overgrown plants or low trees, etc. Have them walk with you starting from the area that a bus or car would drop you off. This gives you a huge advantage when you start your classes and have to negotiate a campus crowded with students.

This is another one of the times you should play the "blind card." If you don't have a friend to help, call the office of special services and see if there is someone who could lead you around until you get the hang of the campus. They would also know the ins and outs of the campus, such as where the restrooms, bookstore, cafeteria, and billing office are located. They have hired people to help you, so take advantage of it.

If it is a new workplace you need to become comfortable with, ask your new boss or the HR person to give you a tour of the office so they can point out things like the lunch room, the conference room, the restrooms, the exits (in case of emergency), and all other pertinent points of interest.

Carrying a backpack of some kind is also a good idea. This helps you keep track of your things more easily. If you have books to carry, a backpack is a great idea, and a fanny pack may be the best choice for your valuables. You don't have to worry about setting things down and leaving them somewhere.

Tip: Learn to keep a mental map of your destinations while you are out walking. This comes in handy if you use a guide dog. Although guide dogs are intelligent, they cannot read your mind and rely on you to know where you are going.

Guide dog is a myth. A guide dog does not watch the traffic light to see when it turns green; you need to listen to the flow of traffic and determine when it is safe to cross a street. It is true that once you take your dog to a location, it is easier for him to take you back to your original starting point because you have dropped skin cells all the way and he can smell his way home. This seems strange, but it is true.

Tip: Do you know what truncated domes are? Not many people do. They are the little bumps on the sidewalk in front of your favorite store. You may have thought they were to keep the carts from rolling into the parking lot, but they do much more than that. They were put there to assist people using a cane. When you feel those bumps with your cane, it is like Braille (although they don't really spell anything) on the ground to alert you to the fact that you are about to step into traffic. In any public place and at crosswalks, you will find these on the ground to warn you. Now you can educate all your friends on what "truncated domes" are, and don't step out into the traffic until you know what is coming at you.

Trick: If you are a woman, you should get a handbag that goes over your head so you can carry it close to your body. It is very easy for someone to steal a handbag from you if he realizes you cannot see well. Someone can run up to you and snatch your bag from your hand before you even know what has happened. This happened to a friend of mine. She had her hand through the handle and inside of her coat pocket. The thief ripped it away, hurting her hand in the process. He was gone and over a fence before she knew it.

Check your area for low-cost transportation. You may have a Dial a Ride type of system that you can use if you fill out an application and get authorization from your doctor that you are legally blind. They can take you from door to door within your town.

Another source is Catholic Charities. They provide rides for those who can no longer drive to get to appointments or even shopping areas. Call your local Catholic church for this information or contact your own religious affiliation to see if they have volunteers who would be willing to provide transportation to you periodically.

It is also a good idea to become familiar with your local bus route. You can call and get a schedule for the busses in your town or county and learn to travel to shopping areas and doctor appointments on your own. Please see the chapter on traveling by yourself before you take the bus by yourself.

Taking Public Transportation

Taking a city bus can be a daunting experience, even if you are fully sighted. If you are trying to get on the right bus, transfer to the next, and then make sure you get off at the right stop without sight, it can be downright scary. I would not suggest that you try this for the first time without a sighted guide.

This is the type of training that would be included in mobility training, and I would highly recommend it to you. Ask your department of rehab to provide this type of training for you. Until you get the training, here are a few suggestions:

- If you will be taking the same bus each day to work or school, have the sighted guide go with you the first and maybe even the second time. Have him or her show you right where the bus stops and find some landmarks to help you make sure you are in the correct spot to board the bus. Make sure you have the correct change or ticket and try to personally meet the bus driver. If you can befriend him or her, it will take you a long way toward your goal, assuming that your goal is to become personally independent and be able to go places by yourself, without a sighted guide.

- Count the number of stops until your stop so you won't be surprised when your stop comes up. You can ask the driver to notify you of your stop, but it doesn't always mean he will remember. He has lots of responsibilities to manage as a driver.

- Make sure that you know the path from the bus stop to the door of your employment or school. Be aware of any changes in the road or construction that might present a problem for street crossing. If you always cross the same street each day and there is no audible signal at that intersection, contact your city to see if it would be possible to install one. Many times, all it takes is a request from someone who frequents that intersection for them to do the installation. The key is to always ask questions and be aware of how you can navigate safely. When VIPS opened its second location, I noticed city workers at the corner so I inquired as to what they were doing. They informed me that they were redoing all of the signals on that street. I asked if they could include an audible signal, and they said they would look into it. They did, and it was installed in a few months later when they revamped all the lights. All I did was ask.

Recently, one of the instructors emailed me that there was a very large pothole in the crosswalk near the corner of the VIPS training facility, right where he crossed the street each day. I called the city, and the next day, it was fixed. I made them aware that several blind persons have to cross there each day and they got right on it.

Be very diligent about knowing the people around you. Keep your valuables close to you and use that backpack or over-the-head handbag so you can keep items secure. You might want to wear a whistle around your neck in case you need to blow it in an emergency.

Tip: Don't lend things to people on the bus. A friend of mine with low vision lent a cell phone to a woman on the bus. When he went to use his phone when he got home, he noticed that it didn't work. She had switched his with one that looked just like his but was broken. You just never know what might happen. People can, and will many times, take advantage of your vision loss.

Most communities have a bus that will transport the elderly and disabled citizens from one point to another for a relatively low cost. Call your city to see what type of transportation is available to you. You might think that it is beneath you to ride such a bus, but once you realize that it is a great step to your independence, you will take advantage of it. You will need to fill out an application and have your doctor sign it to prove that you are legally blind. Some communities require that you take the city bus, unless you are unable to navigate the bus system, then you can ride the door-to-door type bus. You have to call several hours or even days ahead to make an appointment for transportation, but it is well worth it to be picked up and dropped off door to door. No city bus will do that.

Just because a door-to-door bus is picking you up, it doesn't mean that the driver is familiar with what a visually impaired person needs. He or she needs to walk you to the door and make sure you enter safely. We had one occasion where a driver simply opened the bus door, sent the blind person out, and left. He was left crying on the sidewalk, not knowing how to get to the door of the center. This is totally unacceptable, and you need to be your own advocate in educating such a driver how you need to be served. Be firm but polite to them. Remember you are an advocate for the whole blind community and part of your responsibility is to educate people about blindness.

Tip: Understand directions to the places you like to go to. In other words, ask questions when people are taking you somewhere. Always know where you are in relation to your home so if you do get separated from your guide, you will be able to tell someone else how to get you back to your home. This includes Dial a Ride bus drivers and taxi drivers. Many times these drivers are new to the area and don't know how to navigate a town. You can be a great help if you can tell them, "Take the first right on Main Street and the second left on

Jackson. The place I am going to is the third house on the right side: 1803 Jackson."

Tip: Always have your identification with you. You may not have a driver's license anymore, but you can get an ID card from the DMV. You will need this at any airport for identification.

Trick: In airports or train stations, there is assistance available. Talk to the person who takes your ticket to arrange for this service. They will get you through security with ease too. You won't have to worry about losing things on the conveyor belt, including your shoes! I have noticed that persons without a driver's license and only a personal identification card draw the attention of the security team, so it is much better that you have an airport employee escorting you so you don't have to be subjected to more scrutiny as you go through the security check. (This tip was from Tim, one of the newest support group members, who had just gone on a trip by himself and was very happy with the assistance.)

Tip: When staying in a hotel, use the door lock and do not open the door to anyone you do not know. If someone comes to your door, ask who it is before you open the door. You might also want to inquire at the check-in desk if there is assistance available to you, should you need it to navigate the hotel premises.

Tip: If you have about eight hundred dollars or so, you could look into an Ultracane. Go to www.ultracane.com to see what is being developed in Europe for the blind. This cane uses sonar similar to what a bat uses to detect things in front of them. It could be an exciting development, although it's a bit expensive now.

Tip: The government has a plan to give everyone a cell phone. If you are on disability, you can get a free phone with unlimited talk and text. Talk to your rehab center or go to www.budgetmobile.com/california. Everyone should feel safe when they are alone and carry a cell phone with them. You can also use it for shopping lists, names and addresses, navigation around town, and accessing the Internet. You can also listen to music on your phone. It can be very dangerous to be out and not have a cell phone to be able to connect with someone if you get in trouble. Don't take the chance. Take the free phone.

Tip: When getting into a car, ask the driver if you can open your own door. This way, you will know exactly where the door is and you can follow the contour of the car to know where the seat is. You feel much more in control.

10

Eating in a Restaurant

There is no question that going to a restaurant is a bit daunting when you can't see your surroundings. Most restaurants are dimly lighted and not prepared to deal with visually impaired customers. They might have a Braille menu, but then, you probably have not learned Braille yet. You could ask them if they have a large print menu, if that helps you. Take a magnifier with you if that helps. (See chapter 21 for sources for magnifiers.)

You literally have to be the one to educate waitresses and waiters to help them serve you better. If you have one restaurant that you frequent, ask for the same waiter or waitress when you check in. They should be able to seat you in that waiter's (or waitress's) station. Slowly teach them what you need to be able to communicate your needs clearly with them.

Start by telling them that you are visually impaired. Don't be demanding, but let them know that you may need a little more help than the average customer. If you are with someone, the waitress or waiter may tend to look to the other person for your order. Simply let them know that you will be ordering for yourself. If you are alone, ask the waitress to read the parts of the menu to you that you are most interested in. If you are with someone, ask him to read the menu to you and then tell him that you will order for yourself.

Tip: Ask the waitress to have the kitchen cut your salad pieces smaller so it will be easier to handle. You might also ask to have it put in a bowl as opposed to a plate. It is much easier to eat from a bowl without accidently pushing it off of a flat plate.

Trick: Use a piece of bread to push food onto your fork. Even sighted people use this trick, so don't be embarrassed when you use it. It is one of the most helpful tools to making sure you can get your food on the fork and into your mouth. After all, if you are spending good money for restaurant food, you want to make sure it all goes into your mouth and not onto the table, your clothes, or the floor.

Tip: Ask them to let you know when they place your water glass on the table and where it is in relation to your plate.

Trick: Be friendly with your waitperson and teach them this trick so they can use it again on another customer. Ask them to verbally tell you where each food is on your plate in relation to a clock. They should be able to tell you, "Sir, your steak is at 3:00, your potatoes are at 6:00, and your vegetable is at 9:00." This helps you not to be completely surprised when you finally put your loaded fork into your mouth.

Tip: If you are by yourself, try to have cash to pay with. Learn to fold your bills so you can identify the denominations easily. This will prevent you from letting the waitress or waiter take your charge card out of your presence and photocopying the number. Just be wise and safe with your charge cards.

11

Magnifying the World around Me

There are many types of magnifiers in the world. Just because it magnifies, doesn't mean it will work for you. Every eye condition will require a different type of device to magnify print on a page. You have to try different ones to find the right one for you. Below are several options that may work for you.

- Closed-circuit TV (CCTV) reading machines. There are many brands of machines out there, and this is something you can research with your eye doctor, the department of rehabilitation, or your local visual impairment center. This type of machine allows you to put any type of reading material on the table and then magnify it to as large as you wish. You could end up with one letter filling the whole screen if that is what you need. You can also change the contrast from a white background with black words to a black background and white words. This is much easier for some visually impaired persons to read.

- Dome magnifier. This is a dome-shaped device that magnifies up to six times. They come in different strengths in glass or acrylic and can be purchased from a map-reading company.

- Handheld magnifiers. These are magnifiers with a handle attached to them. These come in all strengths and some come with lights built into them. This is helpful to some and not helpful at all to others. Try them out before you buy. They come in all strengths of magnification.

- Electronic magnifiers. These are handy for reading mail, catalogs, books, or price tags in your favorite store. You can place it over a tag, freeze it, and then bring it up to your eye to see what it has recorded. You can change the magnification to whatever strength you need. These devices can be expensive to purchase, so you might investigate eBay to see if you can find a used or refurbished one at a discounted price. You may be able to use your smartphone like this with a purchased app. Check with your phone carrier to see what apps are available for this purpose.

12

Organizing My Home

Before you lost your sight, you may have been a clean freak or maybe you were a bit messy when it came to housework. When your sight is diminished, you will find that if you don't put everything in its place, you won't be able to find it again or you may fall over it.

Another reason to keep things organized is for your own safety. Leaving a cabinet door open or not putting away a step stool can be a disaster waiting to happen. If others live with you, make sure they know to push their chairs in after they pull them out from the table.

Pets are another concern. Dogs and cats usually don't know to avoid you in your own home. They might lie down right in front of you and trip you when you get up. One of the support group members was just sent to the emergency room for lots of bumps and bruises after she fell over her friend's dog. She was on her way out the door to take an eight-hour bus drive and had to do it in a lot of pain. Make sure the pets are secure when you are navigating through your own environment or visiting a friend.

Paperwork is something that can get away from you when it is difficult to see what is on each paper. Try to keep it organized by never just putting it down on the table to be dealt with later. When the mail comes, put it in a bill-paying drawer, file it in the proper category, or throw it into the trash. This will prevent you from collecting junk mail and accidently mixing it with important papers.

If need be, ask a friend or relative to help you read and pay your bills. Many times bills can be paid over the phone. You may want to talk with your bank to see if you can arrange for automatic transfers and deposits. This will eliminate trips to the bank.

Identifying Bill Denominations

Everyone needs to carry a certain amount of cash. Change is pretty easy to identify by size, but bills are another story. There are methods of identifying your bills and you will have to decide what method you would like to use.

There are devices called "bill identifiers" that will help you identify each denomination verbally. Purchase these in one of the catalogues listed in chapter 21 or try http://www.bep.gov/uscurrencyreaderpgm.html to get a free one from the Bureau of Engraving and Printing. There is an online application for you to get one free that includes audio instructions on how to use it.

Trick: You can also learn to fold your money so you can identify it easily in your wallet.

- Leave one-dollar bills unfolded.
- Fold five-dollar bills lengthwise.
- Fold ten-dollar bills by width.
- Fold twenty-dollar bills lengthwise and then by width. Or you can fold them just lengthwise and put them in a separate section of your wallet.

Tip: If you take a bus or cab and know the exact amount of money you will need each time, put it in a designated wallet or envelope that you can identify easily. This will keep you from having to figure out bill denominations on the spot. It just makes sense not to take your wallet out in public and flash your money around. There are people who will take advantage of the fact that you cannot see and could rob you or pick your pocket.

Housecleaning Tips from an Independent Living Instructor

Keeping your home clean is obviously going to be a bit more difficult without good eyesight. Reaching around and behind the toilet has never been fun for me, and I have pretty good eyesight. So attempting to clean areas you cannot see will be a real challenge. Many people are leery of reaching into those areas, fearful that there might be a bug there or something sharp sticking out that could hurt them. Short of hiring a full-time housecleaner, you will need to learn to do it yourself.

There are methods of cleaning so as to maintain a clean and germ-free environment for you and your family, so I recommend you follow the advice of Roxann, who is an independent living instructor. Her first piece of advice is to relax and not try to do everything in one day. Learn to do a little at a time, and soon you will gain the confidence to do what you need to do to maintain an organized home.

Kitchen countertops. Before cleaning a countertop, run your hand over the entire area carefully to feel if there are any large pieces of food or liquid left on it. This will prevent smearing things around the countertop. Remove items off of the countertop and put them in a safe place. Clean the counter with a rag and mild soap and then dry it with a towel. Feel it again to make sure there are no sticky spots and return the items.

Floors. Start in the corner and work your way out of the room. Go back and wipe it with a towel to dry it.

Refrigerator. You may want to purchase some inexpensive, vinyl placemats to line the shelves of your refrigerator. When a spill happens, you can simply remove the placemat and wash it. This is much easier than trying to reach into the refrigerator to clean up a sticky mess.

Toilets. You might think this is gross, but you need to clean toilets with your bare hands. It is very hard to feel things with gloves on. You can use a Mr. Screen to clean the ring out. You can purchase these at a hardware store, and they are very effective on toilet stains. Don't use bleach because it could splash out and you might not see where it goes. It will remove the color in a rug or your clothes. Don't forget to wipe around and behind the toilet.

Bathroom sinks and countertops. Make sure everything is off of the countertop. Spray with a cleaner, and clean with rag. Dry off. Don't forget the mirror, even if you don't look into it. Replace items on the counter.

Tubs and showers. I know you are not used to feeling the tub and shower for dirt, but if you do, you will notice that soap scum is easy to feel. Spray it down with cleaner and wipe clean, and then dry. If you squeegee the shower walls each time you shower, they will stay clean longer.

Laundry. Learn how to pour out your laundry soap in the proper amounts for your wash. Separate the colors; use a color identifier if you need to. Put identification pins on items that match. If you buy colored socks, try to get ones with different textures so you can match them up properly.

Dusting. When you dust your home, be sure to remove items from each surface and place them in a safe place. Dust thoroughly and then return the items. Don't forget the tops of cabinets and low spots.

Vacuuming. Make sure that all items are picked up from your carpet before you vacuum. Small toys don't do well in a vacuum.

There are lots of ways to organize your home so you can find things when you need them.

Tip: As soon as something new comes into your home, put it away, throw it away, or give it away. This will go a long way in keeping you organized.

Tip: Go through your kitchen cupboards and get rid of items you are not going to be using. You want as little as possible in your cupboards so things are easier to find.

Tip: PenFriend. This handy little item gives you the ability to mark things with a small dot that contains a memory chip of some type. You place it on the item, hold the tip of the pen to the dot, and audibly record your voice to document the contents. For instance, you may have a pill bottle that has instructions on it for daily use. Simply place the dot on the bottle, touch it with the PenFriend, and say, "Aspirin: take one capsule with meal, three times a day. Call pharmacy at 444-4444 for refill. Prescription number is 550001. Primary doctor is Doc Holiday at 555-4000." This will assure you don't take the wrong thing at the wrong time and you will be able to refill your prescription when needed. This item can be ordered on Amazon or in one of the catalogs listed in the chapter on finding specialty items.

Tip: CD collections can be identified with the PenFriend.

Trick: Use rubber bands around items to identify them. For instance, if you have one lipstick you like more than others, put a rubber band around it to identify it among the others in your purse.

Tip: Buy hard plastic cups to replace your glass ones. You can get great-looking acrylic drinking glasses that won't shatter if they are knocked off of a table. Trust me: it will happen and you don't want to have to clean up broken glass with partial or no sight.

Tip: Buy a liquid measure indicator. This is a little device that you put at the top of a coffee cup or other container to let you know when the liquid reaches the top. The other alternative is to stick your finger in the cup, and that can be painful if it is hot water. (See chapter 21 for resources for this item.)

Trick: When doing your laundry, put a safety pin on matching clothes like a blouse and pants. If you have more than one outfit that matches, pin a button on them.

Tip: When you need information, call the library and ask the reference librarian to look up what you need. That is their job, and they are very happy to do so.

Tip: Put dividers in your clothes drawers so you can find socks, etc.

Tip: When traveling, use separate ziplock bags for underwear and socks.

Trick: Roll PJs up for both travel and at home. This will help you identify them from clothes.

Tip: If you take pills at each meal, use a tiny dipping bowl to put them in. This way, they won't roll out on the floor and get lost.

13

Preparing and Cooking a Meal

Many people who were used to cooking before they lost their sight are hesitant to go back into the kitchen after they have lost a significant amount of their vision. This fear is completely understandable, as the kitchen holds potential dangers when knives and heat are involved; it isn't impossible though. There are many tips and tricks that can be applied to help the visually impaired person feel confident in his or her kitchen again.

As I have mentioned before, this is an area where VIPS does a lot of training. One of the instructors is completely blind from birth, and another is losing a little more sight each year. They are both fully capable of teaching anyone to gain the confidence they need to feel comfortable in their own kitchen. I have included some great recipes in this chapter that Roxann teaches in her classes. I hope you will gain the confidence to try one or two. Her clients always enjoy the process, and the staff usually benefits from the results that are left over.

If you don't have access to this type of training, I will attempt to give you as many tips as I possibly can to ensure your safety as you adjust your cooking techniques to compensate for your vision loss. Since everyone has different tastes, you should adjust your menus to your own family.

When learning cooking skills, it is important to know how to cook the things you really want to eat. Knowing how to make scrambled eggs isn't really important if you and your family are allergic to them, so don't waste time learning that skill. You will need to learn to crack an egg and get it into a bowl, how to dispose of the shells properly, and how to know if you dropped shells in your eggs. These are skills you will need to know for cooking and baking lots of dishes.

If you are a diabetic, please learn to cook the foods that will help you maintain a healthy blood sugar level. Take it one meal at a time, and soon you will be back to cooking all the things you used to cook when you were fully sighted.

Below are a few tips from the support group members.

Tip: Whatever you are cooking, learn to move things to the back of the counter so you don't knock them onto the floor. If you are going to boil noodles, turn the water on to boil and set the noodles to the back of the counter to wait for the water to boil. This will give you more room to work on your other dishes.

Tip: If you have people other than your family over for, say an iced tea, before they leave, ask them for their glass. This will prevent you from knocking it over later when you have forgotten that it is there. Your family should be expected to put their glasses into the sink so you don't knock them over.

Tip: You can purchase finger guards that fit over your fingers so you can't cut them when slicing vegetables, fruits, or anything you might want to cut with a sharp knife.

Tip: Purchase heatproof gloves that fit like gloves but won't allow you to be burned when you take out a pan from the oven or pull the rack out. These come in fabric or silicone material. I do need to tell you that the fabric ones do not work if they get wet. Make sure you keep them dry before grabbing onto a hot pan. The silicone ones will work wet or dry.

Tip: Purchase a level indicator to put into a cup to let you know when it is almost full. Place it on the side of the cup. Carefully pour the liquid into the cup and it will beep when the water hits the appropriate level. (These can be purchased in the catalogs mentioned in chapter 21.)

Tip: You can purchase measuring spoons and cups with tactile lines on the sides to indicate the amount of the measurement. (Purchase in the specialty items catalog mentioned in chapter 21.)

Tip: Purchase a tray with sides to put your cutting board on. This way, if you are cutting something and it falls off the board, it will be contained on the tray and not roll away. You could use a cookie sheet with sides for this also.

Tip: Place bump dots on the strategic points on your oven temp gauge, dishwasher, microwave, clothes washer and dryer, etc. This will make it easier for you to find, "Off," "Bake," "Wash," etc. Order these in the catalogs suggested in chapter 21.

Tip: When preparing a salad, put the dressing in a separate dish so you can add what you want or dip your salad into it.

Tip: Put dividers in your kitchen drawers, and don't mix knives with other utensils.

Tip: Freeze bread to make peanut butter sandwiches with. The peanut butter will spread much easier and won't tear the bread.

Tip: There is a glove called a fillet glove that is used to cut fish. You can put this on your left hand, if you are right handed, when you cut anything. This has steel in the fabric and will protect you from cutting your left hand.

Tip: Use a spatter guard on your frying pans to keep from getting spattered. This lets the steam out but not the grease spatters.

Tip: Measuring out a teaspoon of vanilla or spices or things like lemon juice can be difficult. VIPS recommends that you purchase a set of metal measuring spoons so they can be bent and used like small scoops. Buy small plastic or glass containers (with lids) with wide mouths so that you can pour your liquid flavorings or spices into them and then use the scoop measuring spoons to retrieve the correct amount for your recipe. For dry ingredients, scoop out and then run your finger across the top to even out the amount. For liquids, simply dip it in and it will fill to the top. Have your cooking bowl close, and carefully transfer the contents to your other ingredients.

You can mark each container with Braille or use a PenFriend to mark it. See chapter 21 to order a PenFriend.

Tip: Bacon is more easily cooked in the oven than on the stove. Spread it on a cookie sheet lined with foil and bake it in the over at 350 degrees for fifteen to twenty minutes or until it is as crispy as you want it to be. Remove with tongs and drain on paper towels.

Recipes That Are Taught to Blind Students

The below recipes were given to me by Roxann Keys, an independent living instructor.

Pepperoni Pizza Pasta Recipe

Prep: 20 minutes
Bake: 20 minutes plus standing

Ingredients
- ✓ 1 1/2 cups uncooked elbow macaroni
- ✓ 2 eggs, lightly beaten
- ✓ 1/3 cup grated Parmesan cheese
- ✓ 1/4 cup sour cream
- ✓ 1/2 teaspoon Italian seasoning
- ✓ 1 1/2 cups pizza sauce (I use a 14-ounce or 16-ounce jar.)
- ✓ 2 cups (8 ounces) shredded part-skim mozzarella cheese
- ✓ 40 slices pepperoni cut in quarters
- ✓ 1 can (2 1/4 ounces) sliced ripe olives, drained

- Cook macaroni according to package directions; drain. Stir in the eggs, Parmesan cheese, sour cream, Italian seasoning, pizza sauce, olives, pepperoni, and cheese, leaving just enough to sprinkle on top. Transfer to a greased 11-inchx7-inch baking dish. Bake at 375 degrees F for 25 minutes. Let stand for 10 minutes before serving.
- **Yield:** 6 servings

Taco Biscuit Bake

Preheat oven at 375 degrees F.
Bake for 20 or 25 minutes until cheese is melted.

Ingredients
- ✓ 1 pound ground beef
- ✓ 2/3 cup water
- ✓ 1 envelope taco seasoning
- ✓ 2 tubes, 12 ounces each, refrigerated buttermilk biscuits
- ✓ 1 can chili with beans
- ✓ 1 cup shredded cheddar cheese
- ✓ Olives can be added if you wish.

Instructions
- Brown the hamburger and drain. Stir in water and taco seasoning. Bring to a boil and cook for about 3 minutes until it begins to thicken.
- Add chili with beans and stir.
- Cut all biscuits into quarters. Place them in the bottom of a 9x13 dish.
- Place beef and chili mixture on top of biscuits, then cheese on top of beef and chili mixture.
- Bake at 375 degrees F for 20 to 25 minutes or until cheese is melted and biscuits are baked.

Bake this about 22 minutes at the longest.

Chicken Noodle Casserole

Preheat oven at 350 degrees F.
Bake for about 25 minutes or until it sounds bubbly.

Ingredients
- ✓ 2 chicken breasts baked or boiled. If baked, season and bake at 350 for 20-25 minutes.
- ✓ 8 ounces egg noodles or a four-cup measuring cup filled to the top.
- ✓ 2 cans cream of chicken soup
- ✓ 1 cup cheddar cheese
- ✓ A few peas if desired, or chopped broccoli is always good.
- ✓ 1/2 role of finely crushed Ritz crackers if desired.

Instructions
- Bake or boil chicken. If you bake, do so at 350 degrees F for about 20 minutes, depending on size.
- Boil noodles according to package and rinse.
- Mix soup, cheese, and peas or broccoli with noodles.
- Dice up chicken and add to noodle mixture.
- Spray an 8x8 casserole dish with nonstick cooking spray and add noodle mixture.
- You can cover with finely crushed Ritz crackers if you wish and then pour a tablespoon of melted butter over top. If you don't put the crackers on, cover and bake. Do not cover if you use crackers.

If you wish to make a 9x13 dish of this, just use 3 or 4 chicken breasts, depending on size, a 16-ounce bag of noodles, and 3 cans of cream of chicken soup. 1 cup of cheese, peas, or broccoli if you wish, and 1 role of crushed Ritz crackers.

Quiche

- ✓ 1 large box of hash browns, 8 paddies.
- ✓ Place in 9x13 dish sprayed with nonstick cooking spray, making sure that they are slightly thawed so you can make even and push them together.
- ✓ Melt 1 cube of butter or margarine and pour over hash browns. Bake at 425 degrees F for 20 minutes.
- ✓ 1 green bell pepper chopped and cooked in microwave
- ✓ 8 leaves spinach finely chopped
- ✓ 1 pound bacon cooked crisp (See cooking instructions below.)
- ✓ 3 1/3 cups grated Swiss cheese
- ✓ 1 1/2 cups grated cheddar cheese
- ✓ 8 eggs, beaten well
- ✓ 2 3/4 cups milk
- ✓ 1 tablespoon hot sauce, beaten well

- When hash browns are out of the oven, sprinkle bell pepper, spinach, bacon, and both cheeses on top.
- Pour egg and milk mixture over the top very slowly so you don't move the cheese.
- Bake uncovered at 350 degrees F for 35 to 40 minutes.

It is easier to prepare this dish if you get your bell pepper, spinach, and bacon cooked and ready. (Some visually impaired people like to cook their bacon in the microwave. Cover it with paper towels to prevent it from splattering the inside of your microwave. If you cook it on the stovetop, you may want to cut it in half to make it easier to flip. You can also cook it in the oven.) I buy my cheese already grated. After that, all you really have to do is get your hash browns cooked and beat up the egg mixture while they are in the oven.

Cream of Broccoli Soup

Ingredients

- ✓ 1 tablespoon butter
- ✓ 1 medium onion(s), chopped (See the finger guards in a catalogue in chapter 21.)
- ✓ 20 ounce frozen, chopped broccoli, thawed
- ✓ 32 1/4 ounce canned condensed cream of potato soup, or 3 (10 3/4) ounce cans
- ✓ 4 cups half and half
- ✓ 1 cup shredded cheddar cheese, sharp
- ✓ 1 tablespoon Dijon mustard
- ✓ 1/8 teaspoon cayenne pepper, or to taste
- ✓ 1 teaspoon kosher salt, or to taste (optional)

Instructions

- Melt butter in a large nonstick saucepan over low heat.
- Add onions and increase heat to medium-low; cover and cook, stirring occasionally, until tender, about 5 minutes.
- Stir in broccoli and potato soup; gradually stir in half and half until blended.
- Increase heat to medium-high and bring to a boil.
- Reduce heat to low and simmer, covered. Stir occasionally, until broccoli is tender, about 10 minutes.
- Remove from heat; stir in cheese, mustard, and cayenne until cheese melts. Season to taste with salt, if desired.
- Yields about 1 1/4 cups per serving. If you simmer the soup longer, it will get thicker and is really good.

Lemon Jell-O Cake

Preheat oven at 325 degrees F.

Bake about 25 to 30 minutes; use toothpick to test.

Ingredients

- ✓ 1 3-ounce package lemon Jell-O
- ✓ 1 lemon cake mix
- ✓ 3/4 cup water and blend
- ✓ 4 teaspoons lemon juice
- ✓ 4 large eggs and blend well
- ✓ 3/4 cup vegetable oil and blend well

- Bake in greased 9x13 pan for about 25 to 30 minutes at 325 degrees F degrees.
- Test with toothpick; toothpick should come out clean.
- While cake is baking, mix the juice of 2 lemons and 2 cups powdered sugar.
- Juice of 2 lemons equals about 6 tablespoons.
- When cake is removed from oven, poke holes all over the top with a fork and pour sugar mixture over the top of the cake.
- Let cool and serve.

Diabetic Recipes

Many people are blinded from the effects of diabetes. If you are a diabetic, you need to learn to cook to help you maintain a healthy blood-sugar level. This includes very few processed foods and lots of vegetables, fruits, and whole grains. All carbohydrates turn to sugar, so try not to eat simple carbs. If you do consume carbs, eat ones with high fiber. These include yams, brown rice, quinoa, etc. Please consult your physician and get professional help with your diet. If you are able to handle a little sugar, here are a few recipes for some desserts that you could try that are under 300 calories. Because you may be the only diabetic in your family, these are recipes for individual servings.

Individual Key Lime Pies

- ✓ 2 heaping tablespoons of Coco Whip. (If your store doesn't have this, you can use sugar-free Cool Whip.)
- ✓ 2 Tablespoon Marshmallow Fluff (Like Jet Puff)
- ✓ 1 Tablespoon lime juice
- ✓ 3 Tablespoon Graham cracker crumbs
- • Stir this together and enjoy your personal pie.

Single S'mores Dessert

These ingredients need to go into a microwavable bowl.
- ✓ 2 heaping Tablespoons of sugar-free Cool Whip
- ✓ 2 Tablespoons of marshmallow fluff
- ✓ 2 Tablespoons of graham cracker crumbs
- ✓ 4 squares organic, dark chocolate (70% or more of cacao)
- • Put in microwave for about 20 seconds. Check and put in for another 10 seconds. When chocolate is soft, stir all together for a melted s'more.

14

Marking My Wardrobe for Color Identification

Knowing what color clothes you are wearing each day is pretty important to most people. Of course, women are usually more concerned with their wardrobe than men, but there are some men who care what they are wearing and want to look good when they go out of their homes.

If you mark your clothing, it will give you much more control over what you pick to wear each day. There are several methods for doing this. You can use safety pins on the hanger to indicate what color it is. You need to make up the key: one for red, two for blue, etc. You may figure out a system that really works for you, so get organizing. You need to know what goes together without asking someone else. Be sure things are not inside out or backward when you put them on. Shoes can be a problem too. You could buy one of those hanging shelves for your closet to store shoes in so you always have two that are the same on your feet. Throwing them in the bottom of the closet just won't work any longer. You just have to be organized.

There are devices that will tell you what color a fabric is just by holding it over the fabric. These are called color identifiers. They can be purchased in one of the specialty items catalogs. (See chapter 21.) They won't tell you if it is a plaid or pattern but may give you several colors that it has identified.

Tip: Put an outfit you like on one hanger. For instance, put a red print blouse with a solid black pair of pants on one hanger. This way, you won't have to search for something to coordinate with your print blouse.

Tip: You could also attach any jewelry you especially like with that outfit to the hanger.

15

Going Shopping in a Store by Myself

Shopping will be a new experience for you. Most likely, you were used to jumping in your car and going shopping whenever you felt like it. Losing your independence by not being able to drive is a difficult pill to swallow. Fortunately, many stores have services to help you with your shopping.

This assistance can be anything from calling in your order over the phone and having items delivered to you to having a personal shopper pick out outfits for you that you can choose from. Simply call the stores you are used to frequenting and ask them what type of services they provide. If your grocery store doesn't deliver, try the one down the street.

When you decide to go to a store, seek out the manager and ask him if he can assist you with your shopping. If you have some sight and have a smartphone, you can keep a list on the phone and then magnify it so you can read it and have it help you find the item. If you are completely blind, take a small recorder with the items you are looking for listed on the recorder. Again, the store might have a service that will gather the items for you, but you will never know if you don't ask.

Asking for assistance is a hard thing to learn for many people. You may have always been the person helping someone else and now you have to ask for help. It is a humbling thing but at this point is a necessary thing. Swallow your pride, and simply ask for help.

My daughter sends her husband to the store where he proceeds to call her, and she then tells him what to purchase and where it is located in the store. She has learned to memorize where things are in her local grocery store. This makes things easy for her husband, who doesn't really care where things are located as long as he can find them quickly. It also prevents them from having to take the girls somewhere they really don't want to be. It is just easier for everyone to do it this way. You will find the right way of doing things in your family with trial and error.

You might really like getting out of the house once in a while. Maybe the grocery store is a safe place for you to explore and learn how to navigate. You just have to find what works for you.

Tip: One of the support group members heard an ad on TV that said, "If you come in to our store and donate to this charity, anything in the store is 30 percent off." She did this, and when she went to buy her favorite perfume, they said that there was a printed disclaimer at the bottom of the TV screen that excluded perfume and makeup. She asked to see a manager and was able to get the 30 percent off because she couldn't see the TV screen. What they said audibly was all she knew: "Anything is 30 percent off."

Learning to purchase things online is a great help. You will need to learn software that reads your computer screen for you before you can start to shop though. Once you do, you can have almost anything shipped right to your door.

16

Entertainment I Can Enjoy

Entertainment for visually impaired persons can sometimes be hard to find. You were probably used to going to the movies, watching television, and going to ball games, plays, or performances. Now that you are not able to see what is happing on a screen or stage, you think it will probably make it more difficult for you to enjoy them as much.

Please don't let your vision limit your socializing. You need to go out as much as you used to and be with people who care about you and enjoy your company. Try to pick things that you enjoy and eliminate the things that are just too hard to enjoy without sight. For instance, I wouldn't pick a foreign film festival, unless you speak the language they are speaking. Subtitles are hard enough to read with good vision and obviously impossible with vision loss. If you pick a movie with lots of dialogue, your friends can fill in the rest for you pretty easily.

Music performances are always a winner. Music is something you can enjoy just as much without sight. In fact, you might want to take up a new instrument at this point in your life. Music can give you great enjoyment, and you really don't need your sight to play any instrument.

One of the support group members was a school music teacher when she lost a significant portion of her sight due to macular degeneration. She did stop teaching in schools but continues to teach private lessons. She also enjoys playing for herself and for support group. She can play by heart almost any song you can think of.

When attending any type of performance, you should play the "blind card." Many venues keep open seating for special circumstances. Also, if it is difficult to navigate in the dark, with steep steps, they may be more than willing to give you front seats.

When my daughter was small, we took her to see Disney on Ice. If we had not made a request, we would have been seated somewhere that would have made it impossible for her to see anything. But we did inquire about special seating for visually impaired persons and were seated in the front row! This changed what could have been a frustrating evening into a beautiful memory for my daughter to cherish forever.

Tip: Call ahead to see if they will make accommodations for low-vision patrons.

Have you thought of trying something like miniature golf? My legally blind daughter beat her husband at miniature golf, causing him to give up the golfer dream. It is really pretty difficult to mess up and lots of fun to try. Don't limit yourself before you even try something new.

How about bowling? Many of our blind citizens are on a blind bowlers team. There are several levels for play. You can bowl just like you did when you were sighted, or they can put up rails that help guide the ball toward the pins. It is great fun and good exercise for everyone, and they even let sighted people on their team. It is all about having a good time with friends.

Tip: One of the support group members and board members, Marty loves to bowl and says it is one of the things he looks forward to each week. He has been completely blind his whole life. He is hoping to bowl 300 each time he goes. He knows he probably won't, but he likes to dream that he could do it and knows that it is possible. He just looks forward to the chance to try each week.

I happened to be at the bowling alley just this week and noticed that the blind bowlers were there. They were having a great time giving it their best shots, mingling with friends, and eating all the wrong things like we all do. They said they wouldn't miss is for the world. I even saw a few strikes!

17

How to Keep Laughter in My Life
(Contributed by Chris Hansen)

Chris Hansen has been blind since birth but has the most cheerful attitude of anyone I know. He always has a smile on his face and has a very strong faith. He offered to contribute to this book, and I quickly accepted. He has authored several books himself and is a prolific poet and a fine musician. He wants to help all visually impaired persons keep laughter in their lives in spite of their sight loss. Enjoy!

Learn to Laugh!

Let's be honest. Those of us who are blind don't know whether to laugh or cry sometimes! Humor often comes out of tragedy. It really is okay to go through a grieving process, but as this book mentions, don't get stuck there. When the sense of loss begins to fade a bit, what do we do? Take a hard look at your life, and something very bittersweet will begin to happen. You'll begin to understand that in the midst of sorrow, there is a real sense of the truly hilarious! If you've lived with blindness for any length of time, you will just begin to smile as you walk down memory lane. Let me share a few very funny stories from my own life, and you will begin to "see" why.

A Prank at a Bank!

Those who know me at all have found out that my sense of humor is somewhat twisted! Years ago, I had a sweet golden retriever guide dog that wouldn't hurt a fly. So one day, I went into my bank, and the lady behind the counter says, "How do you know if I'm giving you the right denominations of money?"

This is where the story takes on a truly twisted turn! So I say to her, "Well, I have this attack dog that has been trained to read denominations, and if you give me the wrong ones, he'll jump up and bite you in the throat!" Surely, I thought, she won't believe such an outrageous story, but what do I know? The story gets better!

My dog was hidden under the counter, so she couldn't even see that I had a dog! So she says, "I don't believe you! You don't even have a dog!" Suddenly, with wicked clarity, I realize that she can't see my dog! So in my most mischievous voice, I say, "I wouldn't bet on that!" Then, in a classic prank, I tell my dog, "Come here! Hop up!" I slap the counter, and up comes my dog! He sticks his face over the counter and nuzzles the face of the teller, who then begins to scream very loudly!

We're not done yet! Other tellers who watched all the fun, and who knew my dog and me, rush over to stem the panic! They grab her foot to prevent her from pushing the alarm summoning the FBI! It turns out she was a brand-new teller who hadn't met me yet! The tellers, in the midst of their laughter, attempted to explain why they had to stop her from summoning the authorities! Just imagine me calling my wife and telling her from jail, "Honey, I can explain!" As you pick yourself up from the floor, prepare yourself! I have more stories to tell.

Better Stop Rushing

Again thinking of the days when I had a guide dog, I remember a day when I rushed into the restroom with my dog and got inside the stall. His tail and my masculine shoes could clearly be seen under the door. In came all these people, but their voices sounded way too high to be men! This was awkward! So I waited for what seemed forever. When all the chatting ladies finally left, I slunk out of the restroom, hoping that no one saw me!

Oh, and there was the time I rushed into a bathroom during an intermission at a concert. (Seems like I rush a lot.) I used what I thought was a urinal, delighted that there wasn't much of a line. Guess that was wishful thinking and I should have known it was too good to be true at an intermission. I reached out to flush and grabbed a faucet! Why on earth didn't some nice gentleman stop me from humiliating myself!

More about dogs. Then there was the time I was a counselor at a youth camp and a boy had taken my guide dog for a walk. The boy and dog were across from me on the other side of a shallow pond. When I needed him again, I called the dog to come to me, thinking surely the dog would go around the water! The boy hung on desperately so as not to lose the running dog who took a straight line right through the pond to get to his master! So there we were—wet dog, wet boy, and counselor—laughing hysterically, and the dog is thinking, *What? You told me to come, right?*

The Vanishing Mobility Student!

I was training at the Orientation Center for the Blind in Albany, California. My mobility instructor dropped me off and said, "Find your way back by any means necessary." He expected me to ask for directions or figure out what direction I was walking by the traffic or the slope of the hill and so forth.

I went into a bakery and asked where I was. In the shop, there happened to be a very nice lady with a few kids and a big station wagon parked out back. She offered me a ride. I thanked her kindly and took her arm as we went out of the back of the bakery to her car.

Meanwhile, my mobility instructor was waiting out front for me to emerge and begin my quest to go back to the school. Well, he waited, and waited, and waited! I, however, had gotten back to the school and was sipping coffee when he finally walked in!

He said, "What happened to you? Weren't you supposed to find your way back?"

I stated what I thought was pretty obvious. "I did find my way back. I got a ride."

"Is that what you would normally do to find your way back?" he asked.

"Sure! If a nice lady with kids offers me a ride, I take it!"

He wasn't very amused. The fact is I did have to redo the assignment and really find my way back by myself.

A Funny Thing Happened at the Theater

A lot of funny things happened at the theater! When I was in junior high and senior high, I was in a theater group for blind and partially sighted kids. Here are a few stories about weird things that happened.

In *Finnegan's Rainbow,* my scene was to play the part of a leprechaun looking for the pot of gold that Finnegan had stolen. So there I was, skipping across the stage. Finnegan heard me coming and prepared a nice Irish greeting.

Well, things didn't go exactly as planned! I skipped over to him and stomped right on his foot! He didn't even miss a beat and in great pain and in a loud voice said, "God be with ye!"

I whispered, "I'm sorry!" Then I say my next line. "God and Mary be with ye!"

Then, somewhat calmer, he responded, "God, Mary, and Joseph be with ye!" And the lines went on like that as I responded, "God, Mary, Joseph, and Jesus be with ye!"

Then there was the production of *Fiddler on the Roof.* The first scene has a dance number where we were singing about

"Tradition"! As I danced in a circle, holding hands with the other dancers, a hand grabbed my foot and moved it!

So back stage, a partially sighted girl approached me and said, "Hey, I grabbed your foot because you were about to step into the foot lights!"

During the same performance, the ghost of the butcher's dead wife was supposed to come swooping onto the stage from behind the curtain; she swooped all right! Actually, she got wrapped up in the curtain and some technicians had to quickly untangle her so she could perform her big scene! Just remember swooping through the air can be hazardous without sight.

I can't forget the time I played the crazy student in *Fiddler on the Roof.* I had a romantic scene that was supposed to be interrupted by the gruff father. So there I went, strolling across the stage to my girl, but I kicked the wooden milk pail she was sitting by. I pretended not to notice as the wooden pale rolled noisily across the wooden stage until a stage hand quickly ran across the stage to grab it before it rolled into the audience!

You know what? Embarrassing moments or not, theater was really good for me! It taught me self-confidence, and it taught me not to worry about the funny stuff. I also learned that what embarrasses you today makes a delightful story tomorrow!

Bouncing Baby Girl

Let me share one of the most terrifying moments of my life as a young and blind dad. My baby daughter needed a diaper change. I put her on the changing table, and for just a moment, I turned around to toss her disposable diaper in the pail behind me.

Mind you, it was just a moment, but it was one moment too long! I heard a horrible thud! I quickly grabbed at the table and she was gone!

I knew in a split second what had happened. She had rolled off the table! For about five seconds, I heard no crying! Those five seconds seemed like an eternity! I thought, *Oh no! She's dead!*

Then I heard the best sound ever! She screamed at the top of her voice! Was I ever glad! So why is this funny? Well, I discovered to my delight that babies really do bounce! Kids manage to bounce back even when we mess up and we think we haven't done the best job as new parents.

Tutor Turned Gymnast

There have been times in my life when I have been employed. I got a job as a tutor helping kids do their homework while their mom took time to fix dinner. One day, I made my young student a ridiculous promise. "If you get all your spelling words right, I'll stand on my head!"

I had written them down in Braille so I could quiz her. Boy, was she motivated! She desperately wanted to see if I would really stand on my head. I thought, *Surely she will miss just one or two words!*

She didn't! She got all twenty words right, which she had never done before. So I emptied my pockets of keys, wallet, and change and placed them on the table. I bent over as she suddenly had a change of heart. "Oh no, Mr. Hansen. You don't have to do this!"

I explained, "No, I am your teacher and I want you to know that you can trust me to keep my word." So down went my head and up went my feet, when the worst of all possibilities happened. In came her mother!

From my gymnastic position, I heard, "What's going on in here!" With my head down and my feet up, I sheepishly explained, "I can explain this! Really, I can!" The girl was laughing hysterically and the mother said, "Oh, this ought to be good!"

This Tastes Terrible!

I pride myself on being a pretty good cook. When my kids were little, they would have agreed. So what a surprise I got one day! I was cooking my famous chicken and rice and gravy. I lightly salted the chicken thighs with garlic salt. I baked them gently at 350 degrees Fahrenheit for about an hour until the skin was nice and crispy. I put four cups of water in a pan and brought it to a boil. Into this I placed the chicken juices and the cut-up pieces of chicken.

I reached into the cupboard and got out a box of rice. I shook the box. It rattled like rice is supposed to. Can you guess where this story is going? Well, you'd be right! I put in the "rice" and stirred for a bit, put a lid over it, turned off the stove, and waited for my masterpiece to be ready in about seven minutes.

I served it with my usual flourish, knowing how much everyone would love my creation. One of my daughters, never shy about her opinion, said to me, "Dad! This tastes terrible!" I was stunned! So with growing curiosity and dread, I took a bite from my plate and—wow! Was she right! It really did taste terrible!

So I got down the box of "rice" and asked with bated breath, "What's in here?" After an awkward pause, my daughter said, "Uh, Dad?" Impatiently, I said, *"Okay! What's in this box?"* Then after another awkward pause, she answered, "Uh, Dad? It's Grapenuts cereal!"

I found out that it isn't enough to listen to the box. I now taste a bit of everything from every box. Had I done that, I would have known it wasn't actually rice. It's a great story to share, and it shows people that we can and should just laugh at ourselves. Others want to laugh but are too polite to laugh out loud. So let's laugh out loud for them!

Perfect Timing

Before the days of smartphones, I had a talking watch that had a rooster sound for an alarm. Okay, you're thinking ahead! I was in church listening to a sermon about the time Jesus told Peter, "Before the rooster crows twice, you shall deny me three times!"

I know what you're thinking, and yes, I did exactly what you're thinking! Just as Jesus was quoted, I pressed the rooster button, and when the rooster crowed on cue, there was suddenly this awkward silence all around me! I thought it was quite appropriate for the moment. I guess I am a bit of a rabble-rouser.

Sometime Things Happen at the Worst Time!

Speaking of church, there I was in the choir with my choir robe on. I had put my talking watch in my pocket under my robe. However, I forgot to turn off the talking voice that announced each hour! Worst of all, I was standing right under an overhead microphone! It was designed to let the whole two thousand people in the auditorium hear everything on stage. And oh boy, what they heard!

We were just about to start one of our songs when the unthinkable happened. My watch announced, "It's eleven o'clock!" The microphone picked up the clear voice, and I heard it broadcast through the big speakers all over the auditorium!

Oh, and then there was the time I got home from choir only to discover that I had worn one black shoe and one brown one!

And then there was the time we were walking down the back stairs of the choir loft and my hand brushed against a light switch. The choir director said, "Chris! Don't even think about it!" One of the men reminded me that this would have plunged the stairs into total blackness! Hey, no problem for me, right?

Let's Get the Poor Blind Man a Wheelchair!

My wife and I had lots of fun on our honeymoon cruise to the Caribbean. We toted lots of souvenirs and luggage too. So there we were at the airport, trying to figure out just how to schlep all of our stuff to our flight.

Along came a well-meaning attendant who said, "Sir, do you need a wheelchair?" I was annoyed and thought, *Well, just because my eyes don't work doesn't mean that my legs don't work!* I was just about to tell him firmly, "No, thank you!"

Then I stopped myself and rethought my whole situation. I mean I had a large amount of luggage to haul, didn't I? And he did bring a wheelchair, didn't he? So my wife, who had the very same idea, said, "Oh, just what we needed!" My wife tossed all sorts of suitcases on the wheelchair and the attendant who was thoroughly embarrassed started pushing the wheelchair, which I obviously didn't need to sit in, through the airport!

What did I do? Well, there I was, proudly walking behind the wheelchair while smiling as if to say, "See? Blind people can walk! But the wheelchair is just what we needed!"

Well, you get the idea. Funny stuff just seems to happen to us!

Below are a few tips to keep the laughter flowing.

Tip: Love! Live! Laugh!
Love: Yes, you are missing your eyes, but you're not missing the rest of life so love what's left of your life.
Live: Your vision is dead or dying, but you're not. So live!

Laugh: Yes, you do feel like crying sometimes, but there are also very funny things that happen all around you, so laugh!

That's why my tip is really three in one. Here it is again: Love! Live! Laugh!

Here are a few other books that Chris Hansen has authored:

- *Revelation Revisited.* A wild trip through John's visions of the end of the world.
- *Secret of the Psalms.* The life of Jesus was predicted in amazing detail a thousand years ahead in the book of Psalms.
- *Grandfather's Journal.* A tender story about a boy who loses his fear of death and learns how to laugh again.

18

Where Will My Strength Come From?

You will no doubt feel like your strength is being drained by your loss of vision. It takes a lot more energy to get tasks done with low or no vision. You may feel like you take one step forward but then take two steps backward. Don't lose heart.

Hopefully, you have loved ones around you to help you with your transition to functioning successfully in an unfamiliar world. They can offer assistance to get you to classes or training that will help you gain your independence once again.

But sometimes, you don't have family or friends to support you in this way. Finding a group of people who are going through the same thing you are going through can be a vital lifeline for you at a time like this. That is why it is so important to join a support group in your area. I cannot emphasize this enough. Pick up the phone, and find help.

If you are already involved with a church, call to let them know your situation. That is what they are there for. If you don't acknowledge the fact that you need outside help, they will never know how they can help you. There are a lot of people out there who are willing to come alongside you and assist you in any way they can.

Your spiritual strength is definitely a vital part of your recovery. You are going through something that has rocked your world and probably shaken you to the core. It is understandable if you are upset with the circumstances and even angry at the world.

More often, when something like blindness hits, people get angry with God. If we have been exposed to teaching about God in our lifetime, we understand that he is powerful, omnipotent, all knowing, and able to do miracles. It is hard to understand, when a tragedy hits, why he would allow or cause something so heinous to happen in our lives. Doesn't he say he loves us?

Getting hit with blindness can often be the catalyst to push us to investigate who this God we really thought we knew is. Have we only taken the word from others about who he is, or do we know him personally and have we put our trust in his Son, Jesus Christ, to lead the way? The Bible says that we can know him personally, so it seems like there is no better time, if we haven't done it before, to investigate that relationship than in the midst of a calamity.

When my daughter was born with an eye disease, I went through all the stages of denial, anger, and depression. We didn't really know what she would be able to see or not see, but we did know that she would never see like other children did and would be prevented from participating in many things that other children could do easily. We lived with uncertainty about her future and the reality of the present, which meant surgery every six weeks and lots of crying and discomfort for her. It is very hard to be handed a child after surgery with large eye patches covering half of her face and told, "Now don't let her cry; it will raise the pressure in her eyes to a dangerous level again." All you can do is cry along with her and walk her for hours on end.

I only tell you this to let you know that I understand a little bit about what it means to question God. I had been raised a Christian and had basic understanding about who he was, but I had never met him personally and didn't really understand how he works in this lifetime. When this all happened, I only knew that I couldn't do it by myself; I needed God to get me through it. He not only got me through it, he gave me life where there was death and completely changed my life.

As the years have gone by and I have seen what a beautiful, talented woman my daughter has become, God's purposes have become clearer to me. I don't know if I would have pursued a close relationship with Jesus had I not had that experience in my life. I would have thought that I had created this little girl and that her father and I would shape her into the woman we wanted her to be. In reality, she belongs to God, and he is very capable of shaping her into what he wants her to be. He knew what we needed and what she needed to become a whole person.

I encourage you to go on your own journey of spiritual growth. Reach out to God, and he will be there for you. Jesus left us a very important message in Revelation 3:20. "Here I am! I stand at the door and knock. If anyone hears my voice and opens the door, I will come in and eat with him, and he with me."

19

Seeking a Higher Education or Employment

There is no reason you should not seek a higher education if you are seeking to better your economic situation and be released from depending upon SSI for your limited income. Everyone wants to feel useful, and if you are of working age, you will no doubt want to work in some capacity. There are avenues to investigate that can help you to achieve your goals both educationally and professionally.

In chapter 2, I gave you the suggestion to contact your state department of rehabilitation. The state is eager to get dependents off the state rolls and will help you achieve your educational goals with employment as the ultimate goal of your endeavors. They may make you jump through some hoops to get some help, but don't give up. If you have a vision center in your area, ask them for an assessment of your condition and for help with applying at the state level. They will help you through the process. The state wants you to be employed, and it is directed to give you the training to make that happen, so take advantage of it.

Tip: Contact your advisor at the local junior college to see what services might be available to you, such as readers, transportation, and scholarships.

Tip: If you don't know how to use a computer with adaptive software that will allow you to see the text greatly magnified or hear the text read to you, you need to learn. This is one of the classes at the center in Modesto. Your state department of rehab can schedule you for classes. Otherwise, it is pretty difficult to get schoolwork done.

Blind People I Know with Successful Careers

You don't need to settle for the myth that there are no careers out there for the blind. In an economy that doesn't offer enough jobs even for the well educated and fully sighted, it is a bit more difficult, but it is possible to have a career if you are determined. After meeting lots of people who have become blinded and had to change careers or stop working altogether, I can assure you that having a good job is what most people seek. No one really wants to sit home and just collect disability. Having a reason to get up each day is very important, and you don't want to get into the habit of not caring about yourself or others. Keep a routine and make a reason to get up and out each day.

All of these people are either legally blind or completely blind:

- professional singer
- telephone solicitor
- instrument musician
- employment manager
- writer
- motivational speaker
- teacher
- salesperson
- business owner
- radio personality

I want to introduce you to a few of my friends who have successful careers in spite of their poor vision or complete blindness. They have succeeded because of their reliability, adaptability, tenacity, and desire to achieve at their jobs. I am not using their full names to protect their privacy.

BN: Bree is blind in one eye and partially sighted in the other. She has two college degrees. She has worked as a CFO for a million-dollar opera company and as director of finances for a water company. Now able to work from home, she is CEO of her own music business and runs an online radio station. She is dedicated to helping female music artists with their careers. She cannot drive a car but is able to do the majority of her work from her home computer and phone.

ML: Marty was blinded at birth because the doctors had to put him in an incubator at birth and unknowingly gave him too much oxygen. Even as a young child, he was fascinated with radios, and when he grew up, he attended college, received a degree in communications, and got a job in a radio station as a DJ. He has worked for most of his life as a radio and sports events announcer. He has the voice for radio and uses it well. Today, he and his wife work together to host a traffic report radio show. Marty also serves on the board of directors of VIPS.

JG: Janet was a bank manager in Sacramento, California, for many years. When she started to lose her sight from retinitis pigmentosa, her job became very difficult. She continued to work there for a year or two but her performance level dropped significantly. She finally decided to leave her job and go on disability. It was a hard thing to realize that she couldn't do the job she had been doing for so many years; she needed help. After attending training classes at VIPS and receiving adaptive computer equipment that helped her tremendously, she volunteered to facilitate the support group for several years. She was eventually hired as the HR manager at VIPS. She also serves on the board of directors and is a great asset as she gives her perspective on issues as a visually impaired person. She does a great job and understands what clients are experiencing with vision loss.

RS: Ryan was an elementary school teacher when his sight failed him. He was heartbroken when he had to leave teaching but jumped right into classes at VIPS. His talents were easily recognized as he completed his classes, and he was hired by VIPS to teach "adjustment to blindness" to other newly blinded clients. He can easily relate to the clients and keeps his sense of humor and positive attitude in the way he teaches the classes. His skills as a teacher are very much appreciated, and he is thrilled to be able to continue to teach.

MM: Mauricio was a mailman when he lost his sight. He is very good at computers and took adaptive technology classes at VIPS when he first started losing his vision. After he graduated, he soon became VIPS's trainer for all things technical. He is very knowledgeable and patient with everyone who isn't as technically talented as he is. His services are very much in demand, and VIPS keeps him very busy. With his skills, he could easily transition to a job in technical support with just about any company. While working at VIPS, he also earned a master's degree. Patience and dedication to the clients are what make him so valuable as an employee. He is also an endless source of one-liner jokes. I am sure he could be a standup comedian as a vocation, but he is a bit shy in front of a crowd.

RK: Roxann was blinded at birth from various eye conditions. She has a college degree and is the independent living manager for VIPS. She teaches all of the students how to cook, clean, and keep their homes organized. This has not been her only career. I know that at one time, she was the person responsible for scheduling all appointments for a carpet cleaning company. She is very organized and takes her responsibilities seriously. This is what has helped her keep her jobs and be valued as a contributing employee.

RM: Richard has had an eye condition since he was around fifteen years old. It has left him legally blind.

He came to America with a rock band because he was such a good musician in his twenties. He is now a terrific salesperson in a retail store. He is a very friendly and knowledgeable salesperson who is always happy to help anyone who stops in his store. He uses a CCTV to help him read brochures and uses ZoomText to access things on his computer. He rides his bike to work because he has never been able to drive a car. Nothing holds him back from having a life always full of music and good friends.

All of these people enjoy their jobs, and with the help of a few special aids, they are all very successful at them. Don't tell yourself you can't continue to work if you are not ready to quit. Pick up your life and start adapting things so you can be productive in your area of interest.

20

Giving Back to My Community

Once you have stabilized your life and learned to live with your condition, you need to think about giving back to others. We have found that this is one of the fastest ways to feel better about yourself as you realize that you can't do all the things you used to do. But there is always someone who can use your help. Call your local help agencies to see if you can do something to volunteer. You can start with phone calls or something you feel you could handle. Once you get involved, you will be hooked and be addicted to helping others.

VIPS has one blind person and two partially sighted people on its board of directors. They provide great insight into problems that face the visually impaired that sighted members forget to consider. One of these members takes many hours to call people each week to invite them to the support group and see how they are doing. It is a vital lifeline to clients. Otherwise, they might just decide to stop coming because no one cares about them. He is a great comfort to others and is always willing to talk on the phone or visit anyone who needs encouragement.

At support group meetings, people come up with great ideas to help other blind persons. One member of the group became active in getting the local government to make streets more accessible to the blind. This member, who had only lost his vision a few months ago, came up with a great idea to present to the City of Modesto. He would like to see the city cut a groove along the painted, crosswalk lines at each intersection to help a person using a cane from wandering out of the crosswalk. When taking his first mobility lessons, he was perplexed as to how he should stay within the crosswalk lines if he could no longer see them. He came up with the idea that if he could guide his cane along a grove in the painted line, he would be able to stay within the crosswalk boundaries. He presented his idea to the city council this month. He is hoping that he can get Modesto to be the first of many cities to provide this service for their cane-traveling citizens.

This is the kind of thing you could do in your community if you put your mind to it. This gentleman led a full life before he lost his sight, and he isn't about to give up the good life because he lost his vision. He is making plans to move forward and not to sit and let life pass him by.

Tip: Your local Lions Club is a great place to start. Become a member and get involved with its humanitarian causes. Its members are great advocates for the blind all around the world. They provide free vision screening, recycle eye glasses, maintain an eye bank, and provide education to raise awareness about preventable eye diseases and much more. They are continually raising money to help the blind and visually impaired around the world, and I am sure you could find a place to fit into the organization.

21

Finding Specialty Items to Help
Me Live More Independently

There are several catalogs where you can order specialty items like watches, magnifiers, games, and kitchen utensils. You can also search online to see what is available that will make your daily tasks easier. Certainly, talking appliances, such as coffeepots, clocks, phones, watches, scales, and voice recorders, can be very helpful in your daily living. You can also purchase software to help you with computer accessibility. This is not an exhaustive list, but it will get you started on your journey to finding what you need.

Something I was just introduced to that is extremely helpful is Echo from Amazon. It costs about $160 and with just a voice command of "Alexa," it will tell you the following: information, music, audio books, news, weather, traffic, sports, Bible passages, and jokes. It will set timers for you, play radio stations or podcasts, define the meaning of words, spell words, and more—instantly. Its far-field voice recognition hears you from across the room. Connected to the cloud, it's always getting smarter. It comes with a phone app that you can add more features to. Its 360-degree omnidirectional audio fills the room with immersive sound.

Echo is compatible with select Belkin WeMo ($39) Philips Hue ($60), SmartThings, Insteon, and Wink ($90) connected devices to control lights and switches with your voice. It plays music from Amazon Music, Prime Music, Pandora, iHeartRadio, TuneIn, and more.

Other Great Resources

- ❖ LS&S. 1-800-468-4789 (many items that will help you with daily tasks).
- ❖ MaxiAIDS. 1-800-522-6294 (more items to help you with daily tasks).
- ❖ Independent Living Aids. 1-800-537-2118, www. independentliving.com.
- ❖ PenFriend. www.penfriend.biz.
- ❖ ZoomText. Contact Synapse Adaptive at 1-800-317-9611. http://www.synapseadaptive.com/aisquared/zoomtext_9/zoomtext_9_home_page.htm.
- ❖ Windows X has a feature that is similar to ZoomText. You can enlarge any text to any size. Free with Windows X.
- ❖ Free money identifier. http://www.bep.gov/uscurrencyreaderpgm.html.

❖ Jaws. Contact Freedom Scientific at 1-800-444- 4443, www.freedomscientific.com/Products/Blindness/ JAWS.

❖ SpeakIt. This is a free button that can be installed on your computer. It lets you listen to text instead of reading it. www. https://chrome.google.com/webstore/detail/speakit/ pgeolalilifpodheeocdmbhehgnkkbak?hl=en-US.

Google what you are looking for on your computer, and you will be surprised at what you can find. There are always things being invented that can help the blind. Don't be afraid to try new things that can expand your horizons.

22

Local and National
Resources for the Blind

- Dial 1-408-752-8052 to get lots of free information, including the following:
    - ✓ the phone number of a business (Yellow Pages)
    - ✓ the weather report—local or anywhere
    - ✓ driving directions
    - ✓ traffic reports
    - ✓ movie information
    - ✓ sports reports
    - ✓ stock market reports
    - ✓ horoscopes
    - ✓ the correct time
    - ✓ news
    - ✓ cheap gas in your area

- If you are interested in investigating the newest breakthroughs in eye-disease cures and preventions, please check out www.eyes.arizona.edu.
- This will give you a wealth of information on eye diseases: http://www.eyespecialist.com/florida/research.htm
- If you love to read books, but because of your blindness you can no longer read for long periods or not at all, contact the Library of Congress for recorded books, magazines, articles, etc. It will also provide an MP3 player to play them. www.loc.gov/nls/. Its phone number is 1-800-424-8567.
- If you need a textbook or educational article that is not already recorded by the Library of Congress, this organization will record it for you: Recording for the Blind in New Jersey (www.rfbdnj.org or 1-800-221-4792).
- American Printing House for the Blind also has talking books and magazines. Its phone number is 1-800-223-1839.
- www.bookshare.com is a good resource for free recorded books.
- For national information concerning issues that affect blind persons, contact the American Foundation for the Blind through www.afb.org.
- To contact the Lions club in your area, visit www.lionsclubs.org.
- To investigate obtaining a guide dog, contact the National Guide Dog Foundation through www.guidedog.org.

- Try www.audible.com for a free trial of audio books, music, and more. It is $14.95 a month after the free trial.
- www.allyoucanbooks.com is free for thirty days and then $19.95 a month for over 30,000 free audio books.
- Visually Impaired Persons Support's phone number is 1-209-522-8477 and address is 1409 H St., Modesto, CA 95354.
- California Department of Rehabilitation: www.dor. ca.gov/.

If you live in a different state, contact your state's department of rehabilitation for assistance.

Tips and Tricks
For VIPS
(Visually Impaired Persons)

Ruth McKinsey speaks from experience, as she has raised a daughter who is partially sighted and she has worked with blind and partially sighted individuals for over thirty years. Because of her passion for helping the blind, she has served on the board of directors of the Visually Impaired Persons Support Center in Modesto, California, for twelve years. Closely working with instructors and clients, she has gleaned many tips and tricks that she thinks will be helpful to anyone who has recently become blind or partially sighted.

If you are losing your sight, this book is a great place to start as you follow a proven plan to work toward building a meaningful life without the help of the good vision you have always depended upon. Put your life back on track and explore many new, exciting options.

This book comes with directions to access a *free,* complete MP3 audio version of the book read by the author.

Tip: Yes, you are missing your eyes, but you're not missing the rest of life, so love what's left of your life.

Tip: When getting into a car, ask the driver if you can open your own door. This way, you will be able to follow the contour of the door and know where the seat is. This gives you more control.

Trick: Measure liquids for cooking by putting them in a wide-mouthed jar; bend metal measuring spoons and dip in to draw out.

Printed in the United States
By Bookmasters

Printed in the United States
By Bookmasters